KETO DIET
LOG BOOK & JOURNAL

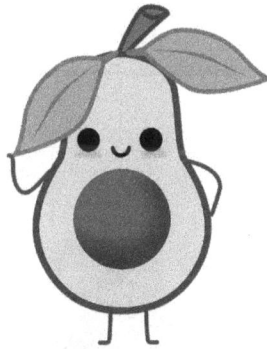

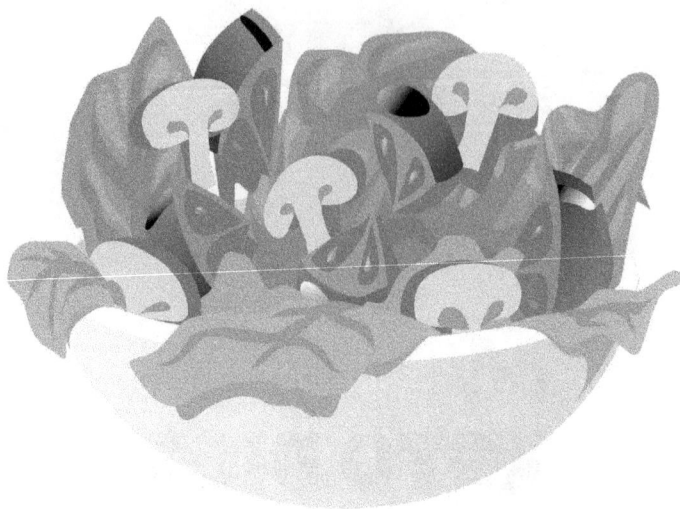

THIS BELONGS TO:

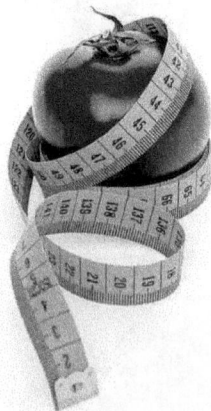

_____

DEDICATION

This **Keto Journal Log Book** is dedicated to all the health conscientious people out there who are wanting to try the Ketogenic Diet & and document their findings in the process.

You are my inspiration for producing books and I'm honored to be a part of keeping all of your Keto notes and records organized.

This journal notebook will help you record your details about your keto journey.

Thoughtfully put together with these sections to record:

Breakfast, Lunch, Dinner, Macrobiotics Tracker, Snacks Tracker, Food Cravings & Fasting, Water Intake, Sleep Tracker, Exercise & Fitness Tracker, How Do I Feel Today, Notes & Comments, and Recipe.

HOW TO USE THIS BOOK

The purpose of this book is to keep all of your Keto notes all in one place. It will help keep you organized.

This Keto Journal will allow you to accurately document every detail about your keto journey. It's a great way to chart your course through ketogenic.

Here are examples of the prompts for you to fill in and write about your experience in this book:

1. ***Goals & Weight*** - Goals you want to achieve, current weight, target weight.

2. ***Breakfast*** - Write what you had for breakfast, tracking macros: protein, fat, carbs, total calories.

3. ***Lunch*** - Log what you had for lunch, tracking macros: protein, fat, carbs, total calories.

4. ***Dinner*** - Record what you had for dinner, tracking macros: protein, fat, carb, total calories.

5. ***Macrobiotics Tracker*** - For recording your amount of protein, fat, carbs & total calories.

6. ***Snacks Tracker*** - List what you had for snacks, tracking macros: protein, fat, carbs, total calories.

7. ***Food Cravings & Fasting*** - Write your food craving & whether you fasted today.

8. ***Water Intake*** - Log your water intake for the day.

9. ***Sleep Tracker*** - Record your hours of sleep.

10. ***Exercise & Fitness Tracker*** - List your exercise & fitness.

11. ***How Do I Feel Today*** - Write how your body is feeling.

12. ***Notes & Comments*** - Blank lined to write anything you wish, for example, your thoughts, your mindset, your motivation, etc.

13. ***Recipe*** - Space for you to write some of your favorite keto recipes at the end of the book.

Enjoy!

GOALS I WANT TO ACHIEVE THROUGH KETO DIET

_____

_____

_____

_____

_____

_____

_____

CURRENT WEIGHT

_____

TARGET WEIGHT

_____

WHAT ARE OTHER THINGS YOU CAN DO TO ACHIEVE YOUR HEALTH GOAL?

_____

_____

_____

_____

_____

_____

DATE: _____   **WEIGHT TODAY:** _____

BREAKFAST	MACROS
	PROTEIN:
	FAT:
	CARBS:
	TOTAL CALORIES:

LUNCH	MACROS
	PROTEIN:
	FAT:
	CARBS:
	TOTAL CALORIES:

DINNER	MACROS
	PROTEIN:
	FAT:
	CARBS:
	TOTAL CALORIES:

SNACKS	MACROS
	PROTEIN:
	FAT:
	CARBS:
	TOTAL CALORIES:

	Y	N		
			WATER INTAKE	
FOOD CRAVINGS			HOURS OF SLEEP	
FASTING DAY			EXERCISE	

HOW DO I FEEL TODAY?

_____
_____
_____
_____

NOTES/COMMENTS

_____
_____
_____
_____

DATE: _____   **WEIGHT TODAY:** _____

BREAKFAST	MACROS
	PROTEIN:
	FAT:
	CARBS:
	TOTAL CALORIES:

LUNCH	MACROS
	PROTEIN:
	FAT:
	CARBS:
	TOTAL CALORIES:

DINNER	MACROS
	PROTEIN:
	FAT:
	CARBS:
	TOTAL CALORIES:

SNACKS	MACROS
	PROTEIN:
	FAT:
	CARBS:
	TOTAL CALORIES:

	Y	N	WATER INTAKE	
FOOD CRAVINGS			HOURS OF SLEEP	
FASTING DAY			EXERCISE	

HOW DO I FEEL TODAY?

_____

_____

_____

_____

NOTES/COMMENTS

_____

_____

_____

_____

DATE: _____   **WEIGHT TODAY: _____**

BREAKFAST	MACROS
	PROTEIN:
	FAT:
	CARBS:
	TOTAL CALORIES:

LUNCH	MACROS
	PROTEIN:
	FAT:
	CARBS:
	TOTAL CALORIES:

DINNER	MACROS
	PROTEIN:
	FAT:
	CARBS:
	TOTAL CALORIES:

SNACKS	MACROS
	PROTEIN:
	FAT:
	CARBS:
	TOTAL CALORIES:

	Y	N		
FOOD CRAVINGS			**WATER INTAKE**	
			HOURS OF SLEEP	
FASTING DAY			**EXERCISE**	

HOW DO I FEEL TODAY?

_____
_____
_____
_____

NOTES/COMMENTS

_____
_____
_____
_____

DATE: _____   **WEIGHT TODAY:** _____

BREAKFAST	MACROS
	PROTEIN:
	FAT:
	CARBS:
	TOTAL CALORIES:

LUNCH	MACROS
	PROTEIN:
	FAT:
	CARBS:
	TOTAL CALORIES:

DINNER	MACROS
	PROTEIN:
	FAT:
	CARBS:
	TOTAL CALORIES:

SNACKS	MACROS
	PROTEIN:
	FAT:
	CARBS:
	TOTAL CALORIES:

	Y	N		
			WATER INTAKE	
FOOD CRAVINGS			HOURS OF SLEEP	
FASTING DAY			EXERCISE	

HOW DO I FEEL TODAY?

_____

_____

_____

_____

NOTES/COMMENTS

_____

_____

_____

_____

DATE: _____ **WEIGHT TODAY:** _____

BREAKFAST	MACROS
	PROTEIN:
	FAT:
	CARBS:
	TOTAL CALORIES:

LUNCH	MACROS
	PROTEIN:
	FAT:
	CARBS:
	TOTAL CALORIES:

DINNER	MACROS
	PROTEIN:
	FAT:
	CARBS:
	TOTAL CALORIES:

SNACKS	MACROS
	PROTEIN:
	FAT:
	CARBS:
	TOTAL CALORIES:

	Y	N		
			WATER INTAKE	
FOOD CRAVINGS			HOURS OF SLEEP	
FASTING DAY			EXERCISE	

HOW DO I FEEL TODAY?

_____

_____

_____

_____

NOTES/COMMENTS

_____

_____

_____

_____

DATE: _____ **WEIGHT TODAY:** _____

BREAKFAST	MACROS
	PROTEIN:
	FAT:
	CARBS:
	TOTAL CALORIES:

LUNCH	MACROS
	PROTEIN:
	FAT:
	CARBS:
	TOTAL CALORIES:

DINNER	MACROS
	PROTEIN:
	FAT:
	CARBS:
	TOTAL CALORIES:

SNACKS	MACROS
	PROTEIN:
	FAT:
	CARBS:
	TOTAL CALORIES:

	Y	N		
			WATER INTAKE	
FOOD CRAVINGS			HOURS OF SLEEP	
FASTING DAY			EXERCISE	

HOW DO I FEEL TODAY?

_____

_____

_____

_____

NOTES/COMMENTS

_____

_____

_____

_____

DATE: _____   **WEIGHT TODAY:** _____

BREAKFAST	MACROS
	PROTEIN:
	FAT:
	CARBS:
	TOTAL CALORIES:

LUNCH	MACROS
	PROTEIN:
	FAT:
	CARBS:
	TOTAL CALORIES:

DINNER	MACROS
	PROTEIN:
	FAT:
	CARBS:
	TOTAL CALORIES:

SNACKS	MACROS
	PROTEIN:
	FAT:
	CARBS:
	TOTAL CALORIES:

	Y	N		
			WATER INTAKE	
FOOD CRAVINGS			**HOURS OF SLEEP**	
FASTING DAY			**EXERCISE**	

HOW DO I FEEL TODAY?

_____

_____

_____

_____

NOTES/COMMENTS

_____

_____

_____

_____

DATE: _____   **WEIGHT TODAY:** _____

BREAKFAST	MACROS
	PROTEIN:
	FAT:
	CARBS:
	TOTAL CALORIES:

LUNCH	MACROS
	PROTEIN:
	FAT:
	CARBS:
	TOTAL CALORIES:

DINNER	MACROS
	PROTEIN:
	FAT:
	CARBS:
	TOTAL CALORIES:

SNACKS	MACROS
	PROTEIN:
	FAT:
	CARBS:
	TOTAL CALORIES:

	Y	N		
			WATER INTAKE	
FOOD CRAVINGS			HOURS OF SLEEP	
FASTING DAY			EXERCISE	

HOW DO I FEEL TODAY?

_____

_____

_____

_____

NOTES/COMMENTS

_____

_____

_____

_____

DATE: _____   **WEIGHT TODAY:** _____

BREAKFAST	MACROS
	PROTEIN:
	FAT:
	CARBS:
	TOTAL CALORIES:

LUNCH	MACROS
	PROTEIN:
	FAT:
	CARBS:
	TOTAL CALORIES:

DINNER	MACROS
	PROTEIN:
	FAT:
	CARBS:
	TOTAL CALORIES:

SNACKS	MACROS
	PROTEIN:
	FAT:
	CARBS:
	TOTAL CALORIES:

	Y	N		
FOOD CRAVINGS			**WATER INTAKE**	
FASTING DAY			**HOURS OF SLEEP**	
			EXERCISE	

HOW DO I FEEL TODAY?

_____

_____

_____

_____

NOTES/COMMENTS

_____

_____

_____

_____

DATE: _____   **WEIGHT TODAY:** _____

BREAKFAST	MACROS
	PROTEIN:
	FAT:
	CARBS:
	TOTAL CALORIES:

LUNCH	MACROS
	PROTEIN:
	FAT:
	CARBS:
	TOTAL CALORIES:

DINNER	MACROS
	PROTEIN:
	FAT:
	CARBS:
	TOTAL CALORIES:

SNACKS	MACROS
	PROTEIN:
	FAT:
	CARBS:
	TOTAL CALORIES:

	Y	N		
			WATER INTAKE	
FOOD CRAVINGS			HOURS OF SLEEP	
FASTING DAY			EXERCISE	

HOW DO I FEEL TODAY?

_____

_____

_____

_____

NOTES/COMMENTS

_____

_____

_____

_____

DATE: _____   WEIGHT TODAY: _____

BREAKFAST	MACROS
	PROTEIN:
	FAT:
	CARBS:
	TOTAL CALORIES:

LUNCH	MACROS
	PROTEIN:
	FAT:
	CARBS:
	TOTAL CALORIES:

DINNER	MACROS
	PROTEIN:
	FAT:
	CARBS:
	TOTAL CALORIES:

SNACKS	MACROS
	PROTEIN:
	FAT:
	CARBS:
	TOTAL CALORIES:

	Y	N		
FOOD CRAVINGS			**WATER INTAKE**	
FASTING DAY			**HOURS OF SLEEP**	
			EXERCISE	

HOW DO I FEEL TODAY?

_____

_____

_____

_____

NOTES/COMMENTS

_____

_____

_____

_____

DATE: _____   WEIGHT TODAY: _____

BREAKFAST	MACROS
	PROTEIN:
	FAT:
	CARBS:
	TOTAL CALORIES:

LUNCH	MACROS
	PROTEIN:
	FAT:
	CARBS:
	TOTAL CALORIES:

DINNER	MACROS
	PROTEIN:
	FAT:
	CARBS:
	TOTAL CALORIES:

SNACKS	MACROS
	PROTEIN:
	FAT:
	CARBS:
	TOTAL CALORIES:

	Y	N
FOOD CRAVINGS		
FASTING DAY		

WATER INTAKE	
HOURS OF SLEEP	
EXERCISE	

HOW DO I FEEL TODAY?

_____

_____

_____

_____

NOTES/COMMENTS

_____

_____

_____

_____

DATE: _____   WEIGHT TODAY: _____

BREAKFAST	MACROS
	PROTEIN:
	FAT:
	CARBS:
	TOTAL CALORIES:

LUNCH	MACROS
	PROTEIN:
	FAT:
	CARBS:
	TOTAL CALORIES:

DINNER	MACROS
	PROTEIN:
	FAT:
	CARBS:
	TOTAL CALORIES:

SNACKS	MACROS
	PROTEIN:
	FAT:
	CARBS:
	TOTAL CALORIES:

	Y	N		
FOOD CRAVINGS			**WATER INTAKE**	
FASTING DAY			**HOURS OF SLEEP**	
			EXERCISE	

HOW DO I FEEL TODAY?

_____

_____

_____

_____

NOTES/COMMENTS

_____

_____

_____

_____

DATE: _____   **WEIGHT TODAY:** _____

BREAKFAST	MACROS
	PROTEIN:
	FAT:
	CARBS:
	TOTAL CALORIES:

LUNCH	MACROS
	PROTEIN:
	FAT:
	CARBS:
	TOTAL CALORIES:

DINNER	MACROS
	PROTEIN:
	FAT:
	CARBS:
	TOTAL CALORIES:

SNACKS	MACROS
	PROTEIN:
	FAT:
	CARBS:
	TOTAL CALORIES:

	Y	N		
			WATER INTAKE	
FOOD CRAVINGS			HOURS OF SLEEP	
FASTING DAY			EXERCISE	

HOW DO I FEEL TODAY?

_____

_____

_____

_____

NOTES/COMMENTS

_____

_____

_____

_____

DATE: _____   **WEIGHT TODAY:** _____

BREAKFAST	MACROS
	PROTEIN:
	FAT:
	CARBS:
	TOTAL CALORIES:

LUNCH	MACROS
	PROTEIN:
	FAT:
	CARBS:
	TOTAL CALORIES:

DINNER	MACROS
	PROTEIN:
	FAT:
	CARBS:
	TOTAL CALORIES:

SNACKS	MACROS
	PROTEIN:
	FAT:
	CARBS:
	TOTAL CALORIES:

	Y	N		
			WATER INTAKE	
FOOD CRAVINGS			HOURS OF SLEEP	
FASTING DAY			EXERCISE	

HOW DO I FEEL TODAY?

_____

_____

_____

_____

NOTES/COMMENTS

_____

_____

_____

_____

DATE: _____   **WEIGHT TODAY:** _____

BREAKFAST	MACROS
	PROTEIN:
	FAT:
	CARBS:
	TOTAL CALORIES:

LUNCH	MACROS
	PROTEIN:
	FAT:
	CARBS:
	TOTAL CALORIES:

DINNER	MACROS
	PROTEIN:
	FAT:
	CARBS:
	TOTAL CALORIES:

SNACKS	MACROS
	PROTEIN:
	FAT:
	CARBS:
	TOTAL CALORIES:

	Y	N		
			WATER INTAKE	
FOOD CRAVINGS			HOURS OF SLEEP	
FASTING DAY			EXERCISE	

HOW DO I FEEL TODAY?

_____
_____
_____
_____

NOTES/COMMENTS

_____
_____
_____
_____

DATE: _____   **WEIGHT TODAY:** _____

BREAKFAST	MACROS
	PROTEIN:
	FAT:
	CARBS:
	TOTAL CALORIES:

LUNCH	MACROS
	PROTEIN:
	FAT:
	CARBS:
	TOTAL CALORIES:

DINNER	MACROS
	PROTEIN:
	FAT:
	CARBS:
	TOTAL CALORIES:

SNACKS	MACROS
	PROTEIN:
	FAT:
	CARBS:
	TOTAL CALORIES:

	Y	N		
			WATER INTAKE	
FOOD CRAVINGS			**HOURS OF SLEEP**	
FASTING DAY			**EXERCISE**	

HOW DO I FEEL TODAY?

_____

_____

_____

_____

NOTES/COMMENTS

_____

_____

_____

_____

DATE: _____   **WEIGHT TODAY:** _____

BREAKFAST	MACROS
	PROTEIN:
	FAT:
	CARBS:
	TOTAL CALORIES:

LUNCH	MACROS
	PROTEIN:
	FAT:
	CARBS:
	TOTAL CALORIES:

DINNER	MACROS
	PROTEIN:
	FAT:
	CARBS:
	TOTAL CALORIES:

SNACKS	MACROS
	PROTEIN:
	FAT:
	CARBS:
	TOTAL CALORIES:

	Y	N		
FOOD CRAVINGS			WATER INTAKE	
FASTING DAY			HOURS OF SLEEP	
			EXERCISE	

HOW DO I FEEL TODAY?

_____

_____

_____

_____

NOTES/COMMENTS

_____

_____

_____

_____

DATE: _____   **WEIGHT TODAY:** _____

BREAKFAST	MACROS
	PROTEIN:
	FAT:
	CARBS:
	TOTAL CALORIES:

LUNCH	MACROS
	PROTEIN:
	FAT:
	CARBS:
	TOTAL CALORIES:

DINNER	MACROS
	PROTEIN:
	FAT:
	CARBS:
	TOTAL CALORIES:

SNACKS	MACROS
	PROTEIN:
	FAT:
	CARBS:
	TOTAL CALORIES:

	Y	N		
			WATER INTAKE	
FOOD CRAVINGS			HOURS OF SLEEP	
FASTING DAY			EXERCISE	

HOW DO I FEEL TODAY?

_____

_____

_____

_____

NOTES/COMMENTS

_____

_____

_____

_____

DATE: _____   **WEIGHT TODAY:** _____

BREAKFAST	MACROS
	PROTEIN:
	FAT:
	CARBS:
	TOTAL CALORIES:

LUNCH	MACROS
	PROTEIN:
	FAT:
	CARBS:
	TOTAL CALORIES:

DINNER	MACROS
	PROTEIN:
	FAT:
	CARBS:
	TOTAL CALORIES:

SNACKS	MACROS
	PROTEIN:
	FAT:
	CARBS:
	TOTAL CALORIES:

	Y	N		
			WATER INTAKE	
FOOD CRAVINGS			HOURS OF SLEEP	
FASTING DAY			EXERCISE	

HOW DO I FEEL TODAY?

_____

_____

_____

_____

NOTES/COMMENTS

_____

_____

_____

_____

DATE: _____   **WEIGHT TODAY:** _____

BREAKFAST	MACROS
	PROTEIN:
	FAT:
	CARBS:
	TOTAL CALORIES:

LUNCH	MACROS
	PROTEIN:
	FAT:
	CARBS:
	TOTAL CALORIES:

DINNER	MACROS
	PROTEIN:
	FAT:
	CARBS:
	TOTAL CALORIES:

SNACKS	MACROS
	PROTEIN:
	FAT:
	CARBS:
	TOTAL CALORIES:

	Y	N		
			WATER INTAKE	
FOOD CRAVINGS			HOURS OF SLEEP	
FASTING DAY			EXERCISE	

HOW DO I FEEL TODAY?

_____

_____

_____

_____

NOTES/COMMENTS

_____

_____

_____

_____

DATE: _____   **WEIGHT TODAY:** _____

BREAKFAST	MACROS
	PROTEIN:
	FAT:
	CARBS:
	TOTAL CALORIES:

LUNCH	MACROS
	PROTEIN:
	FAT:
	CARBS:
	TOTAL CALORIES:

DINNER	MACROS
	PROTEIN:
	FAT:
	CARBS:
	TOTAL CALORIES:

SNACKS	MACROS
	PROTEIN:
	FAT:
	CARBS:
	TOTAL CALORIES:

	Y	N		
			WATER INTAKE	
FOOD CRAVINGS			**HOURS OF SLEEP**	
FASTING DAY			**EXERCISE**	

HOW DO I FEEL TODAY?

_____

_____

_____

_____

NOTES/COMMENTS

_____

_____

_____

_____

DATE: _____   WEIGHT TODAY: _____

BREAKFAST	MACROS
	PROTEIN:
	FAT:
	CARBS:
	TOTAL CALORIES:

LUNCH	MACROS
	PROTEIN:
	FAT:
	CARBS:
	TOTAL CALORIES:

DINNER	MACROS
	PROTEIN:
	FAT:
	CARBS:
	TOTAL CALORIES:

SNACKS	MACROS
	PROTEIN:
	FAT:
	CARBS:
	TOTAL CALORIES:

	Y	N		
			WATER INTAKE	
FOOD CRAVINGS			**HOURS OF SLEEP**	
FASTING DAY			**EXERCISE**	

HOW DO I FEEL TODAY?

_____

_____

_____

_____

NOTES/COMMENTS

_____

_____

_____

_____

DATE: _____   WEIGHT TODAY: _____

BREAKFAST	MACROS
	PROTEIN:
	FAT:
	CARBS:
	TOTAL CALORIES:

LUNCH	MACROS
	PROTEIN:
	FAT:
	CARBS:
	TOTAL CALORIES:

DINNER	MACROS
	PROTEIN:
	FAT:
	CARBS:
	TOTAL CALORIES:

SNACKS	MACROS
	PROTEIN:
	FAT:
	CARBS:
	TOTAL CALORIES:

	Y	N		
			WATER INTAKE	
FOOD CRAVINGS			HOURS OF SLEEP	
FASTING DAY			EXERCISE	

HOW DO I FEEL TODAY?

_____

_____

_____

_____

NOTES/COMMENTS

_____

_____

_____

_____

DATE: _____   **WEIGHT TODAY:** _____

BREAKFAST	MACROS
	PROTEIN:
	FAT:
	CARBS:
	TOTAL CALORIES:

LUNCH	MACROS
	PROTEIN:
	FAT:
	CARBS:
	TOTAL CALORIES:

DINNER	MACROS
	PROTEIN:
	FAT:
	CARBS:
	TOTAL CALORIES:

SNACKS	MACROS
	PROTEIN:
	FAT:
	CARBS:
	TOTAL CALORIES:

	Y	N		
			WATER INTAKE	
FOOD CRAVINGS			HOURS OF SLEEP	
FASTING DAY			EXERCISE	

HOW DO I FEEL TODAY?

_____

_____

_____

_____

NOTES/COMMENTS

_____

_____

_____

_____

DATE: _____   **WEIGHT TODAY:** _____

BREAKFAST	MACROS
	PROTEIN:
	FAT:
	CARBS:
	TOTAL CALORIES:

LUNCH	MACROS
	PROTEIN:
	FAT:
	CARBS:
	TOTAL CALORIES:

DINNER	MACROS
	PROTEIN:
	FAT:
	CARBS:
	TOTAL CALORIES:

SNACKS	MACROS
	PROTEIN:
	FAT:
	CARBS:
	TOTAL CALORIES:

	Y	N		
			WATER INTAKE	
FOOD CRAVINGS			**HOURS OF SLEEP**	
FASTING DAY			**EXERCISE**	

HOW DO I FEEL TODAY?

_____

_____

_____

_____

NOTES/COMMENTS

_____

_____

_____

_____

DATE: _____   WEIGHT TODAY: _____

BREAKFAST	MACROS
	PROTEIN:
	FAT:
	CARBS:
	TOTAL CALORIES:

LUNCH	MACROS
	PROTEIN:
	FAT:
	CARBS:
	TOTAL CALORIES:

DINNER	MACROS
	PROTEIN:
	FAT:
	CARBS:
	TOTAL CALORIES:

SNACKS	MACROS
	PROTEIN:
	FAT:
	CARBS:
	TOTAL CALORIES:

	Y	N		
			WATER INTAKE	
FOOD CRAVINGS			HOURS OF SLEEP	
FASTING DAY			EXERCISE	

HOW DO I FEEL TODAY?

_____

_____

_____

_____

NOTES/COMMENTS

_____

_____

_____

_____

DATE: _____   **WEIGHT TODAY:** _____

BREAKFAST	MACROS
	PROTEIN:
	FAT:
	CARBS:
	TOTAL CALORIES:

LUNCH	MACROS
	PROTEIN:
	FAT:
	CARBS:
	TOTAL CALORIES:

DINNER	MACROS
	PROTEIN:
	FAT:
	CARBS:
	TOTAL CALORIES:

SNACKS	MACROS
	PROTEIN:
	FAT:
	CARBS:
	TOTAL CALORIES:

	Y	N		
			WATER INTAKE	
FOOD CRAVINGS			HOURS OF SLEEP	
FASTING DAY			EXERCISE	

HOW DO I FEEL TODAY?

_____

_____

_____

_____

NOTES/COMMENTS

_____

_____

_____

_____

DATE: _____   **WEIGHT TODAY:** _____

BREAKFAST	MACROS
	PROTEIN:
	FAT:
	CARBS:
	TOTAL CALORIES:

LUNCH	MACROS
	PROTEIN:
	FAT:
	CARBS:
	TOTAL CALORIES:

DINNER	MACROS
	PROTEIN:
	FAT:
	CARBS:
	TOTAL CALORIES:

SNACKS	MACROS
	PROTEIN:
	FAT:
	CARBS:
	TOTAL CALORIES:

	Y	N
FOOD CRAVINGS		
FASTING DAY		

WATER INTAKE	
HOURS OF SLEEP	
EXERCISE	

HOW DO I FEEL TODAY?

NOTES/COMMENTS

DATE: _____   WEIGHT TODAY: _____

BREAKFAST	MACROS
	PROTEIN:
	FAT:
	CARBS:
	TOTAL CALORIES:

LUNCH	MACROS
	PROTEIN:
	FAT:
	CARBS:
	TOTAL CALORIES:

DINNER	MACROS
	PROTEIN:
	FAT:
	CARBS:
	TOTAL CALORIES:

SNACKS	MACROS
	PROTEIN:
	FAT:
	CARBS:
	TOTAL CALORIES:

	Y	N		
FOOD CRAVINGS			WATER INTAKE	
FASTING DAY			HOURS OF SLEEP	
			EXERCISE	

HOW DO I FEEL TODAY?

NOTES/COMMENTS

DATE: _____   **WEIGHT TODAY:** _____

BREAKFAST	MACROS
	PROTEIN:
	FAT:
	CARBS:
	TOTAL CALORIES:

LUNCH	MACROS
	PROTEIN:
	FAT:
	CARBS:
	TOTAL CALORIES:

DINNER	MACROS
	PROTEIN:
	FAT:
	CARBS:
	TOTAL CALORIES:

SNACKS	MACROS
	PROTEIN:
	FAT:
	CARBS:
	TOTAL CALORIES:

	Y	N	**WATER INTAKE**	
FOOD CRAVINGS			**HOURS OF SLEEP**	
FASTING DAY			**EXERCISE**	

HOW DO I FEEL TODAY?

_____

_____

_____

_____

NOTES/COMMENTS

_____

_____

_____

_____

DATE: _____   **WEIGHT TODAY:** _____

BREAKFAST	MACROS
	PROTEIN:
	FAT:
	CARBS:
	TOTAL CALORIES:

LUNCH	MACROS
	PROTEIN:
	FAT:
	CARBS:
	TOTAL CALORIES:

DINNER	MACROS
	PROTEIN:
	FAT:
	CARBS:
	TOTAL CALORIES:

SNACKS	MACROS
	PROTEIN:
	FAT:
	CARBS:
	TOTAL CALORIES:

	Y	N		
			WATER INTAKE	
FOOD CRAVINGS			HOURS OF SLEEP	
FASTING DAY			EXERCISE	

HOW DO I FEEL TODAY?

_____
_____
_____
_____

NOTES/COMMENTS

_____
_____
_____
_____

DATE: _____   **WEIGHT TODAY:** _____

BREAKFAST	MACROS
	PROTEIN:
	FAT:
	CARBS:
	TOTAL CALORIES:

LUNCH	MACROS
	PROTEIN:
	FAT:
	CARBS:
	TOTAL CALORIES:

DINNER	MACROS
	PROTEIN:
	FAT:
	CARBS:
	TOTAL CALORIES:

SNACKS	MACROS
	PROTEIN:
	FAT:
	CARBS:
	TOTAL CALORIES:

	Y	N		
			WATER INTAKE	
FOOD CRAVINGS			**HOURS OF SLEEP**	
FASTING DAY			**EXERCISE**	

HOW DO I FEEL TODAY?

_____

_____

_____

_____

NOTES/COMMENTS

_____

_____

_____

_____

DATE: _____ **WEIGHT TODAY:** _____

BREAKFAST	MACROS
	PROTEIN:
	FAT:
	CARBS:
	TOTAL CALORIES:

LUNCH	MACROS
	PROTEIN:
	FAT:
	CARBS:
	TOTAL CALORIES:

DINNER	MACROS
	PROTEIN:
	FAT:
	CARBS:
	TOTAL CALORIES:

SNACKS	MACROS
	PROTEIN:
	FAT:
	CARBS:
	TOTAL CALORIES:

	Y	N		
			WATER INTAKE	
FOOD CRAVINGS			**HOURS OF SLEEP**	
FASTING DAY			**EXERCISE**	

HOW DO I FEEL TODAY?

_____

_____

_____

_____

NOTES/COMMENTS

_____

_____

_____

_____

DATE: _____   **WEIGHT TODAY:** _____

BREAKFAST	MACROS
	PROTEIN:
	FAT:
	CARBS:
	TOTAL CALORIES:

LUNCH	MACROS
	PROTEIN:
	FAT:
	CARBS:
	TOTAL CALORIES:

DINNER	MACROS
	PROTEIN:
	FAT:
	CARBS:
	TOTAL CALORIES:

SNACKS	MACROS
	PROTEIN:
	FAT:
	CARBS:
	TOTAL CALORIES:

	Y	N		
			WATER INTAKE	
FOOD CRAVINGS			HOURS OF SLEEP	
FASTING DAY			EXERCISE	

HOW DO I FEEL TODAY?

_____

_____

_____

_____

NOTES/COMMENTS

_____

_____

_____

_____

DATE: _____   WEIGHT TODAY: _____

BREAKFAST	MACROS
	PROTEIN:
	FAT:
	CARBS:
	TOTAL CALORIES:

LUNCH	MACROS
	PROTEIN:
	FAT:
	CARBS:
	TOTAL CALORIES:

DINNER	MACROS
	PROTEIN:
	FAT:
	CARBS:
	TOTAL CALORIES:

SNACKS	MACROS
	PROTEIN:
	FAT:
	CARBS:
	TOTAL CALORIES:

	Y	N		
			WATER INTAKE	
FOOD CRAVINGS			HOURS OF SLEEP	
FASTING DAY			EXERCISE	

HOW DO I FEEL TODAY?

_____

_____

_____

_____

NOTES/COMMENTS

_____

_____

_____

_____

DATE: _____ **WEIGHT TODAY:** _____

BREAKFAST	MACROS
	PROTEIN:
	FAT:
	CARBS:
	TOTAL CALORIES:

LUNCH	MACROS
	PROTEIN:
	FAT:
	CARBS:
	TOTAL CALORIES:

DINNER	MACROS
	PROTEIN:
	FAT:
	CARBS:
	TOTAL CALORIES:

SNACKS	MACROS
	PROTEIN:
	FAT:
	CARBS:
	TOTAL CALORIES:

	Y	N		
			WATER INTAKE	
FOOD CRAVINGS			**HOURS OF SLEEP**	
FASTING DAY			**EXERCISE**	

HOW DO I FEEL TODAY?

_____

_____

_____

_____

NOTES/COMMENTS

_____

_____

_____

_____

DATE: _____ **WEIGHT TODAY:** _____

BREAKFAST	MACROS
	PROTEIN:
	FAT:
	CARBS:
	TOTAL CALORIES:

LUNCH	MACROS
	PROTEIN:
	FAT:
	CARBS:
	TOTAL CALORIES:

DINNER	MACROS
	PROTEIN:
	FAT:
	CARBS:
	TOTAL CALORIES:

SNACKS	MACROS
	PROTEIN:
	FAT:
	CARBS:
	TOTAL CALORIES:

	Y	N
FOOD CRAVINGS		
FASTING DAY		

WATER INTAKE	
HOURS OF SLEEP	
EXERCISE	

HOW DO I FEEL TODAY?

_____

_____

_____

_____

NOTES/COMMENTS

_____

_____

_____

_____

DATE: _____   **WEIGHT TODAY:** _____

BREAKFAST	MACROS
	PROTEIN:
	FAT:
	CARBS:
	TOTAL CALORIES:

LUNCH	MACROS
	PROTEIN:
	FAT:
	CARBS:
	TOTAL CALORIES:

DINNER	MACROS
	PROTEIN:
	FAT:
	CARBS:
	TOTAL CALORIES:

SNACKS	MACROS
	PROTEIN:
	FAT:
	CARBS:
	TOTAL CALORIES:

	Y	N		
			WATER INTAKE	
FOOD CRAVINGS			HOURS OF SLEEP	
FASTING DAY			EXERCISE	

HOW DO I FEEL TODAY?

_____

_____

_____

_____

NOTES/COMMENTS

_____

_____

_____

_____

DATE: _____   WEIGHT TODAY: _____

BREAKFAST	MACROS
	PROTEIN:
	FAT:
	CARBS:
	TOTAL CALORIES:

LUNCH	MACROS
	PROTEIN:
	FAT:
	CARBS:
	TOTAL CALORIES:

DINNER	MACROS
	PROTEIN:
	FAT:
	CARBS:
	TOTAL CALORIES:

SNACKS	MACROS
	PROTEIN:
	FAT:
	CARBS:
	TOTAL CALORIES:

	Y	N		
FOOD CRAVINGS			**WATER INTAKE**	
FASTING DAY			**HOURS OF SLEEP**	
			EXERCISE	

HOW DO I FEEL TODAY?

_____

_____

_____

_____

NOTES/COMMENTS

_____

_____

_____

_____

DATE: _____   WEIGHT TODAY: _____

BREAKFAST	MACROS
	PROTEIN:
	FAT:
	CARBS:
	TOTAL CALORIES:

LUNCH	MACROS
	PROTEIN:
	FAT:
	CARBS:
	TOTAL CALORIES:

DINNER	MACROS
	PROTEIN:
	FAT:
	CARBS:
	TOTAL CALORIES:

SNACKS	MACROS
	PROTEIN:
	FAT:
	CARBS:
	TOTAL CALORIES:

	Y	N		
			WATER INTAKE	
FOOD CRAVINGS			**HOURS OF SLEEP**	
FASTING DAY			**EXERCISE**	

HOW DO I FEEL TODAY?

_____

_____

_____

_____

NOTES/COMMENTS

_____

_____

_____

_____

DATE: _____   **WEIGHT TODAY:** _____

BREAKFAST	MACROS
	PROTEIN:
	FAT:
	CARBS:
	TOTAL CALORIES:

LUNCH	MACROS
	PROTEIN:
	FAT:
	CARBS:
	TOTAL CALORIES:

DINNER	MACROS
	PROTEIN:
	FAT:
	CARBS:
	TOTAL CALORIES:

SNACKS	MACROS
	PROTEIN:
	FAT:
	CARBS:
	TOTAL CALORIES:

	Y	N	WATER INTAKE	
FOOD CRAVINGS			HOURS OF SLEEP	
FASTING DAY			EXERCISE	

HOW DO I FEEL TODAY?

_____

_____

_____

_____

NOTES/COMMENTS

_____

_____

_____

_____

DATE: _____   **WEIGHT TODAY:** _____

BREAKFAST	MACROS
	PROTEIN:
	FAT:
	CARBS:
	TOTAL CALORIES:

LUNCH	MACROS
	PROTEIN:
	FAT:
	CARBS:
	TOTAL CALORIES:

DINNER	MACROS
	PROTEIN:
	FAT:
	CARBS:
	TOTAL CALORIES:

SNACKS	MACROS
	PROTEIN:
	FAT:
	CARBS:
	TOTAL CALORIES:

	Y	N		
FOOD CRAVINGS			**WATER INTAKE**	
FASTING DAY			**HOURS OF SLEEP**	
			EXERCISE	

HOW DO I FEEL TODAY?

_____

_____

_____

_____

NOTES/COMMENTS

_____

_____

_____

_____

DATE: _____   **WEIGHT TODAY:** _____

BREAKFAST	MACROS
	PROTEIN:
	FAT:
	CARBS:
	TOTAL CALORIES:

LUNCH	MACROS
	PROTEIN:
	FAT:
	CARBS:
	TOTAL CALORIES:

DINNER	MACROS
	PROTEIN:
	FAT:
	CARBS:
	TOTAL CALORIES:

SNACKS	MACROS
	PROTEIN:
	FAT:
	CARBS:
	TOTAL CALORIES:

	Y	N		
			WATER INTAKE	
FOOD CRAVINGS			HOURS OF SLEEP	
FASTING DAY			EXERCISE	

HOW DO I FEEL TODAY?

_____

_____

_____

_____

NOTES/COMMENTS

_____

_____

_____

_____

DATE: _____   **WEIGHT TODAY:** _____

BREAKFAST	MACROS
	PROTEIN:
	FAT:
	CARBS:
	TOTAL CALORIES:

LUNCH	MACROS
	PROTEIN:
	FAT:
	CARBS:
	TOTAL CALORIES:

DINNER	MACROS
	PROTEIN:
	FAT:
	CARBS:
	TOTAL CALORIES:

SNACKS	MACROS
	PROTEIN:
	FAT:
	CARBS:
	TOTAL CALORIES:

	Y	N		
FOOD CRAVINGS			WATER INTAKE	
FASTING DAY			HOURS OF SLEEP	
			EXERCISE	

HOW DO I FEEL TODAY?

_____

_____

_____

_____

NOTES/COMMENTS

_____

_____

_____

_____

DATE: _____   **WEIGHT TODAY:** _____

BREAKFAST	MACROS
	PROTEIN:
	FAT:
	CARBS:
	TOTAL CALORIES:

LUNCH	MACROS
	PROTEIN:
	FAT:
	CARBS:
	TOTAL CALORIES:

DINNER	MACROS
	PROTEIN:
	FAT:
	CARBS:
	TOTAL CALORIES:

SNACKS	MACROS
	PROTEIN:
	FAT:
	CARBS:
	TOTAL CALORIES:

	Y	N		
			WATER INTAKE	
FOOD CRAVINGS			HOURS OF SLEEP	
FASTING DAY			EXERCISE	

HOW DO I FEEL TODAY?

_____

_____

_____

_____

NOTES/COMMENTS

_____

_____

_____

_____

DATE: _____   WEIGHT TODAY: _____

BREAKFAST	MACROS
	PROTEIN:
	FAT:
	CARBS:
	TOTAL CALORIES:

LUNCH	MACROS
	PROTEIN:
	FAT:
	CARBS:
	TOTAL CALORIES:

DINNER	MACROS
	PROTEIN:
	FAT:
	CARBS:
	TOTAL CALORIES:

SNACKS	MACROS
	PROTEIN:
	FAT:
	CARBS:
	TOTAL CALORIES:

	Y	N		
			WATER INTAKE	
FOOD CRAVINGS			HOURS OF SLEEP	
FASTING DAY			EXERCISE	

HOW DO I FEEL TODAY?

_____

_____

_____

_____

NOTES/COMMENTS

_____

_____

_____

_____

DATE: _____   **WEIGHT TODAY:** _____

BREAKFAST	MACROS
	PROTEIN:
	FAT:
	CARBS:
	TOTAL CALORIES:

LUNCH	MACROS
	PROTEIN:
	FAT:
	CARBS:
	TOTAL CALORIES:

DINNER	MACROS
	PROTEIN:
	FAT:
	CARBS:
	TOTAL CALORIES:

SNACKS	MACROS
	PROTEIN:
	FAT:
	CARBS:
	TOTAL CALORIES:

	Y	N		
			WATER INTAKE	
FOOD CRAVINGS			HOURS OF SLEEP	
FASTING DAY			EXERCISE	

HOW DO I FEEL TODAY?

_____

_____

_____

_____

NOTES/COMMENTS

_____

_____

_____

_____

DATE: _____   **WEIGHT TODAY:** _____

BREAKFAST	MACROS
	PROTEIN:
	FAT:
	CARBS:
	TOTAL CALORIES:

LUNCH	MACROS
	PROTEIN:
	FAT:
	CARBS:
	TOTAL CALORIES:

DINNER	MACROS
	PROTEIN:
	FAT:
	CARBS:
	TOTAL CALORIES:

SNACKS	MACROS
	PROTEIN:
	FAT:
	CARBS:
	TOTAL CALORIES:

	Y	N		
FOOD CRAVINGS			**WATER INTAKE**	
FASTING DAY			**HOURS OF SLEEP**	
			EXERCISE	

HOW DO I FEEL TODAY?

_____

_____

_____

_____

NOTES/COMMENTS

_____

_____

_____

_____

HOW DO I FEEL SO FAR WITH THE KETO DIET?

_____

_____

_____

_____

_____

_____

CURRENT WEIGHT

_____

TARGET WEIGHT

_____

AM I HAPPY WITH THE WEIGHT I HAVE LOST? HOW CAN I BE HAPPIER?

_____

_____

_____

_____

_____

_____

Recipe: _____

Prep Time: _____

Cook Time: _____

Serves: _____

INGREDIENTS

_____ _____

_____ _____

_____ _____

_____ _____

_____ _____

DIRECTIONS

_____

_____

_____

_____

_____

_____

_____

_____

_____

RECIPE: _____

PREP TIME: _____

COOK TIME: _____

SERVES: _____

INGREDIENTS

------------------------ ------------------------

------------------------ ------------------------

------------------------ ------------------------

------------------------ ------------------------

------------------------ ------------------------

DIRECTIONS

_____

_____

_____

_____

_____

_____

_____

_____

_____

RECIPE: _____

PREP TIME: _____

COOK TIME: _____

SERVES: _____

INGREDIENTS

_____ _____

_____ _____

_____ _____

_____ _____

_____ _____

DIRECTIONS

_____

_____

_____

_____

_____

_____

_____

_____

RECIPE: _____

PREP TIME: _____

COOK TIME: _____

SERVES: _____

INGREDIENTS

_____ _____

_____ _____

_____ _____

_____ _____

_____ _____

DIRECTIONS

_____

_____

_____

_____

_____

_____

_____

_____

_____

RECIPE: _____

PREP TIME: _____

COOK TIME: _____

SERVES: _____

INGREDIENTS

_____ _____

_____ _____

_____ _____

_____ _____

_____ _____

DIRECTIONS

_____

_____

_____

_____

_____

_____

_____

_____

_____

RECIPE: _____

PREP TIME: _____

COOK TIME: _____

SERVES: _____

INGREDIENTS

_____   _____

_____   _____

_____   _____

_____   _____

_____   _____

DIRECTIONS

_____

_____

_____

_____

_____

_____

_____

_____

_____

RECIPE: _____

PREP TIME: _____

COOK TIME: _____

SERVES: _____

INGREDIENTS

_____   _____

_____   _____

_____   _____

_____   _____

_____   _____

DIRECTIONS

_____

_____

_____

_____

_____

_____

_____

_____

_____

RECIPE: _____

PREP TIME: _____

COOK TIME: _____

SERVES: _____

INGREDIENTS

_____ _____

_____ _____

_____ _____

_____ _____

_____ _____

DIRECTIONS

_____

_____

_____

_____

_____

_____

_____

_____

_____